SOUTHERN KETO COOKBOOK

The Traditional Comforting Food That You will Love to Lose Weight and Maintain Health with This Perfect Guide of Southern Keto Diet Containin 50+ Classic Recipes fo Beginners.

By

Sophia Moore

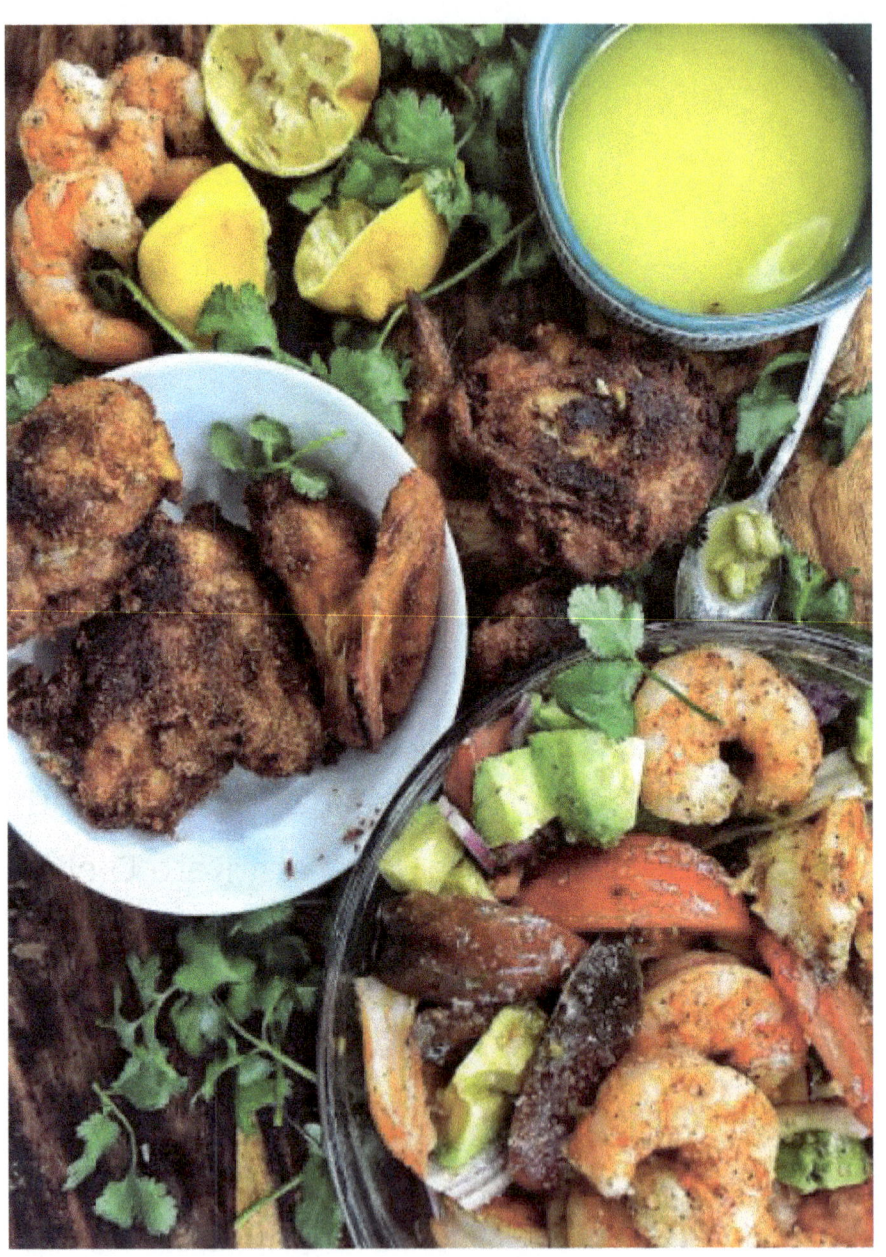

© **Copyright 2021 - All rights reserved.**

The content contained within this book may not be reproduced, duplicated or transmitted without direct written permission from the author or the publisher.

Under no circumstances will any blame or legal responsibility be held against the publisher, or author, for any damages, reparation, or monetary loss due to the information contained within this book. Either directly or indirectly.

Legal Notice:

This book is copyright protected. This book is only for personal use. You cannot amend, distribute, sell, use, quote or paraphrase any part, or the content within this book, without the consent of the author or publisher.

Disclaimer Notice:

Please note the information contained within this document is for educational and entertainment purposes only. All effort has been executed to present accurate, up to date, and reliable, complete information. No warranties of any kind are declared or implied. Readers acknowledge that the author is not engaging in the rendering of legal, financial, medical or professional advice. The content within this book has been derived from various sources.

Please consult a licensed professional before attempting any techniques outlined in this book. By reading this document, the reader agrees that under no circumstances is the author responsible for any losses, direct or indirect, which are incurred as a result of the use of information contained within this document, including, but not limited to, errors, omissions, or inaccuracies.

Table of Contents

INTRODUCTION -------------------------------- **10**

Recipes -- **13**

1. Papa John's Garlic Sauce ---------------------- 13
2. SAUTÉED CABBAGE WITH CUMIN SEEDS ---- 14
3. REFRESHING APPLE-CILANTRO GREEN SMOOTHIE -- 16
4. Buffalo Chicken Wraps ------------------------ 18
5. Pesto Salad ------------------------------------ 20
6. Pan Chicken Curry ----------------------------- 22
7. Pan Chocolate Chicken Mole ------------------ 24
8. Raspberry Sorbet ------------------------------ 26
9. Mexican Coffee -------------------------------- 29
10. Café coffee ----------------------------------- 31
11. Chocolate Orange Coffee with cake ---------- 32
12. Keto Turkey Stir Fry ------------------------- 33
13. Chicken Asparagus Stir-Fry ------------------ 35
14. Sea Bass with Tapenade Cream Sauce ------ 37
15. Keto Chinese Breakfast Chaffle ------------- 40

16. Chicken Bites With Chaffles ------------------42

17. Fish With Chaffle Bites-----------------------44

18. Cheddar & Herb Chaffle (Keto Low Carb) ----46

19. Chaffles With Keto Ice Cream ----------------48

20. Vanilla Mozzarella Chaffles ------------------49

21. Chili's Molten Lava Cake---------------------51

22. Cracker Barrel Banana Pudding --------------53

23. Cracker Barrel Carrot Cake------------------55

24. Cracker Barrel Cherry Chocolate Cobbler ----58

25. Golden Corral Bread Pudding-----------------60

26. Olive Garden Apple Carmelina ---------------62

27. Starbucks Tarragon Chicken Salad -----------64

28. Steak'n Shake Frisco Melt -------------------65

29. Applebee's Garlic & Peppercorn Fried Shrimp 67

30. Applebee's Garlic Mashed Potatoes -----------69

31. Applebee's Tequila Lime Chicken -------------71

32. Buca di Beppo Chicken Marsala ---------------73

33. Buca di Beppo Penne Cardinale ---------------75

34. Buca di Beppo Chicken Saltimbocca ----------77

35. Carino's Angel Hair with Artichokes-----------79

36. Carino's Five Meat Tuscan Pasta --------------81

37. Carino's Grilled Chicken Bowtie Festival------83

38. Cheesecake Factory Jambalaya Pasta --------85

39. Cracker Barrel Baby Carrots------------------87

40. Cracker Barrel Corn Bread Dressing ---------88

41. Cracker Barrel Country Green Beans --------90

42. Cracker Barrel Grilled Chicken Tenders-------91

43. Popeye's Biscuits ------------------------------92

44. Popeye's Cajun Gravy ------------------------93

45. McDonald's Steak, Egg, & Cheese Bagel Sandwich---95

46. Starbucks Bran Muffins ------------------------97

47. Applebee's Pico de Gallo----------------------99

48. Applebee's Spinach & Artichoke Dip -------- 101

49. Olive Garden Pasta e Fagioli Soup ---------- 102

50. Olive Garden Pasta Roma Soup ------------- 104

51. Olive Garden Seafood Pasta Chowder ------ 106

52. Olive Garden Zuppa Toscana Soup --------- 108

53. P.F. Chang's Wonton Soup ------------------ 110

54. Red Lobster Clam Chowder ------------------ 112

55. Ruby Tuesday White Chicken Chili ---------- 114

56. Steak'n Shake Chili --------------------------- 116

57. T.G.I. Friday's Broccoli Cheese Soup ------- 118

58. T.G.I. Friday's French Onion Soup ---------- 119

59. Applebee's Oriental Chicken Salad ---------- 121

Conclusion ---------------------------------------**123**

INTRODUCTION

You all, I am a Southern woman who loves some Southern food, and this book delights you! Get ready because it's page after page of delicious low-carb foods, including many popular Southern-style dishes like cornbread, hash brown casserole, finger sandwiches, baby pups, pie, and more! South Keto cookbook with hash brown casserole in a bowl

Grab the paperback or Kindle edition of the book to join the fun! Tasha struggled with her weight from an early age and put on her first diet at the age of nine. I can totally relate to it; I was put into Weight Watchers at a young age when they told you exactly what you should be eating - I remember that tuna, lettuce, and boiled eggs are always a daily thing.

Being deprived of the foods she wanted and her craving led Tasha to search for those foods when she was not at home. This led to many years of yo-yo dieting, which resulted in her weighing more than 300 pounds. In the end, I came across the keto diet and haven't looked back since!

She's gone from years of yo-yo dieting to a keto lifestyle - and now she's truly living her best life. Tasha's full story in Southern Keto is truly incredible, as she also shares her battle with Crohn's disease and how the Ketogenic lifestyle changed her life. As someone who has suffered from colon cancer, her story is very connected to me. I think you'll be really inspired by Tasha, in addition to falling in love with her delicious and easy recipes.

Eating and keto cooking

Fill in silicone molds with blueberry keto pie mixture
This section provides a helpful list of keto-friendly foods, including essential nutrients, oils, and fats, as well as sweeteners and where to get them. One of the staples that I mentioned keeps in her pantry is oat fiber, which is new to me, and I want to try it. I love that the author includes a list of her favorite kitchen gadgets and gadgets!

Keto practical advice

This Southern keto cookbook is open to beneficial keto food swaps.

This is one of my favorite parts of the book that isn't related to the recipe! In this section, you'll find low-carb trade-offs and suggestions for replacing your favorite high-carb foods with keto-friendly options like replacing toast with low-carb cheese chips. You'll also find ways to do the keto diet on a budget, the keto diet for special occasions, takeout suggestions, and ways to maintain it while you travel.

Recipes

1. Papa John's Garlic Sauce

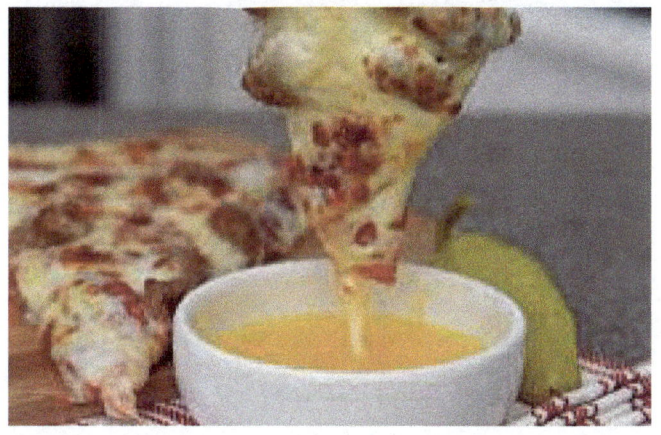

Prep Time: 10 Mins | Cooking Time: 10 Mins | Serve: 2

INGREDIENTS:

- Stick margarine
- ¼ Tsp. salt
- 1 Tsp. garlic powder

DIRECTIONS:

1. Melt margarine in the microwave for about 30 seconds.
2. Add salt & garlic powder to taste.
3. Microwave the mixture for 5 seconds longer.

2. SAUTÉED CABBAGE WITH CUMIN SEEDS

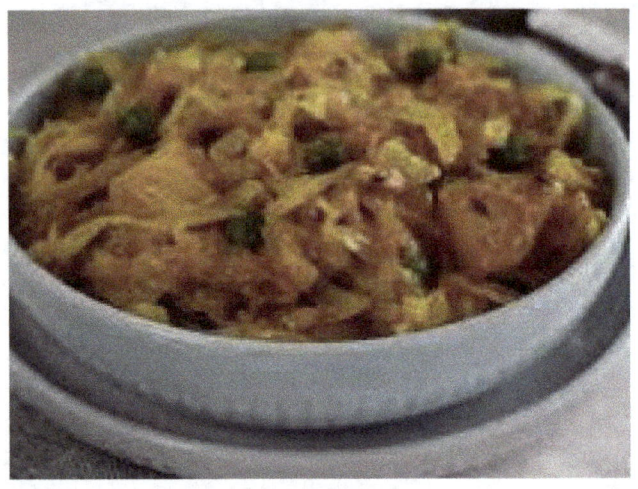

Prep Time: 10 Mins | Cooking Time: 20 Mins | Serve: 2

INGREDIENTS:

- 1 Tbsp. whole cumin seeds
- 1 Tbsp. virgin coconut oil
- 4 cups sliced green cabbage
- Sea salt

DIRECTIONS:

1. Heat an 11- or 12-inch skillet over medium-high heat.

2. Add the cumin seeds & toast them for about 30 seconds.
3. Then add the coconut oil & cabbage & sauté for 4 to 5 min. Season to taste with sea salt.

3. REFRESHING APPLE-CILANTRO GREEN SMOOTHIE

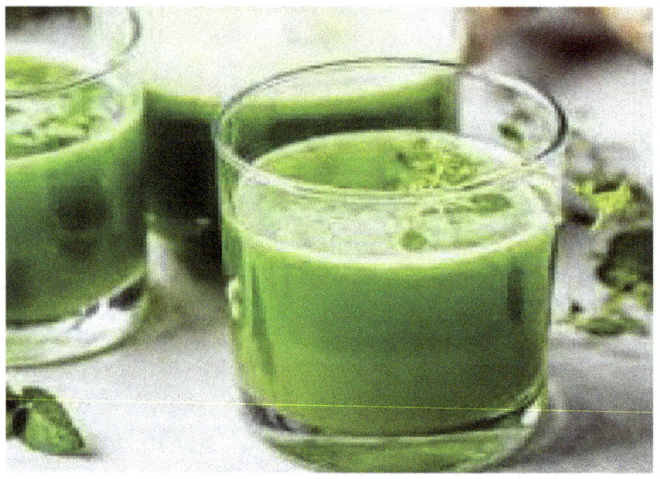

Prep Time: 10 Mins | Cooking Time: 0 Mins | Serve: 4

INGREDIENTS:

- 2 apples, cored
- 2 small avocados
- 4 to 5 collard greens
- 1 bunch fresh cilantro, leaves & stems
- freshly squeezed juice of 2 limes
- 3 cups water

DIRECTIONS:

1. Place all the ingredients into a high-powered blender & blend until smooth.
2. Add more water for a thinner consistency. This smoothie will keep in the refrigerator for up to 2 days.

4. Buffalo Chicken Wraps

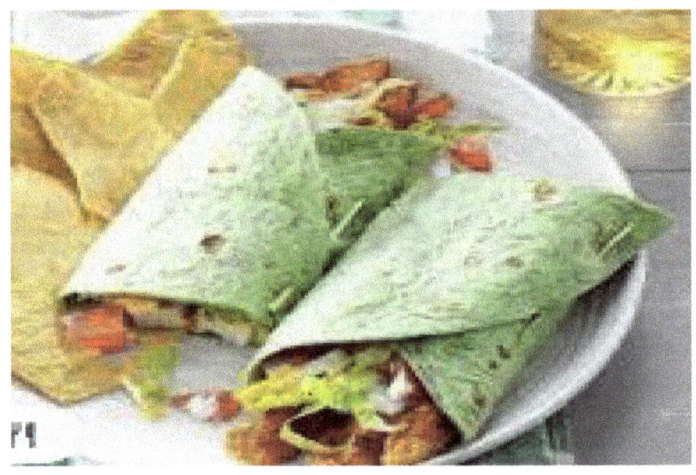

Prep Time: 20 Mins | Cooking Time: 40 Mins | Serve: 3

INGREDIENTS:
- For the chicken:
- 24 oz. boneless skinless chicken breast
- 1 celery stalk
- ½ onion, diced
- 1 clove garlic
- 16 oz. fat-free low sodium chicken broth
- ½ mug hot cayenne pepper sauce
- For the wraps:
- 6 large lettuce leaves, Bibb
- 1 ½ mugs shredded carrots

- 2 large celery stalks, cut into 2-inch matchsticks

DIRECTIONS:

1. Put the chicken, celery stalks, garlic & broth in a pan & cook covered on high for 4 hrs.
2. Remove the chicken & shred it. Retain only half a mug of broth in the pan & throw out the rest. Put the shredded chicken back to the pan with the hot pepper sauce & cook for an extra 30 mins on high. For the wraps, put half a mug of buffalo chicken on each lettuce leaf with ¼ mug of carrots, celery & your favorite dressing & wrap.
3. Serve and enjoy.

5. Pesto Salad

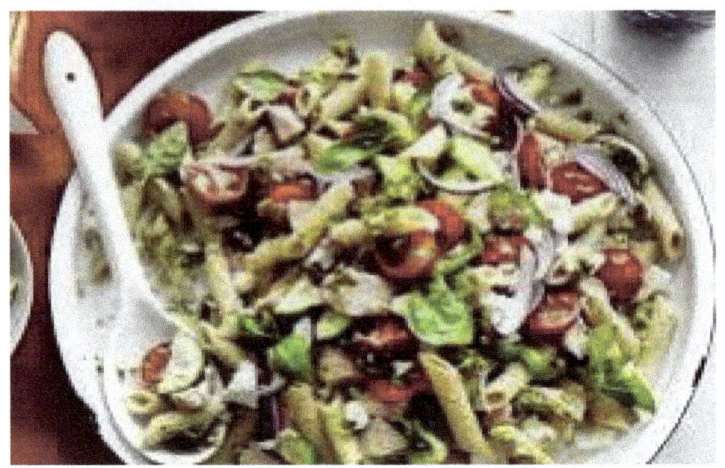

Prep Time: 20 Mins | Cooking Time: 60 Mins | Serve: 4

INGREDIENTS:

- 1.5 lb. organic boneless chicken breasts (3 or 4 pieces)
- 1 garlic clove, chopped ½ white onion, chopped
- 1 mug organic chicken broth ¼ teaspoon garlic powder
- Dash of salt & freshly ground pepper
- Pesto Sauce:
- 1 mug fresh basil
- 1 ½ mug spinach
- ½ mug cashews, walnuts, or nuts of choice
- 1 tablespoon extra-virgin olive oil
- 1 garlic clove

- ½ lemon, juiced
- Dash Himalayan sea salt to taste
- Dash Freshly ground pepper, to taste.
- Dash red pepper flakes
- Additional INGREDIENTS:
- ¼ mug pine nuts

DIRECTIONS:

1. Put the chicken breasts along with the broth in the pan & put in garlic, onion, garlic powder, salt & pepper to it.
2. Cook on high for 3 hrs & then remove the chicken & shred it. For the pesto sauce, combine all the sauce ingredients other than the oil in a food processor & pulse it until it is ground. Put in the oil & pulse again. Combine the chicken & the sauce in a casserole.
3. Toast the pine nuts for around 3 mins in a pan.
4. Top the salad with pine nuts & refrigerate for some time.
5. Serve and enjoy.

6. Pan Chicken Curry

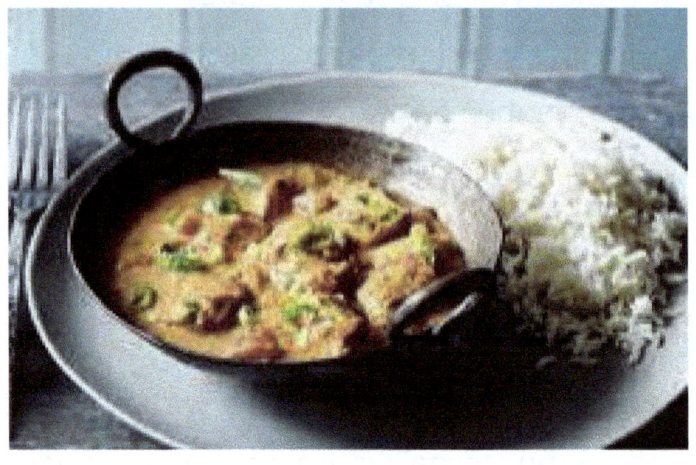

Prep Time: 20 Mins | Cooking Time: 40 Mins | Serve: 3

INGREDIENTS:

- 2 onions, chopped
- 2 tablespoon olive oil
- 2 cloves garlic, crushed
- 2 chickens, diced
- 1 tin (14 oz.) coconut cream
- 1 mug water
- 2 yellow bell peppers, chopped into cubes
- 2 medium yellow squash, chopped into cubes
- 6 tablespoon yellow curry paste
- 2 tomatoes

DIRECTIONS:

1. Brown the onions in a pan with crushed garlic in olive oil.
2. Put all the vegetables in the pan along with the onions & the garlic.
3. Put the chicken in the pan & cook on low for 8 hrs or for 4 hrs on high.

7. Pan Chocolate Chicken Mole

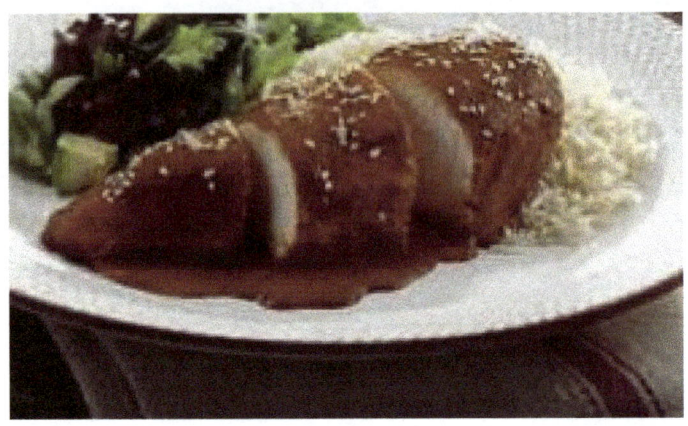

Prep Time: 20 Mins | Cooking Time: 40 Mins | Serve: 3

INGREDIENTS:

- 2 lbs. chicken breasts & legs, bone in, Skin removed
- Salt & pepper
- 2 tablespoon coconut oil
- 1 medium onion, chopped
- 4 cloves garlic, crushed or minced
- 6 - 7 tomatoes, peeled, seeded & chopped
- 5 dried New Mexico chili peppers, rehydrated & chopped
- ¼ mug almond butter
- 2.5 oz. dark chocolate

- 1 teaspoon sea salt
- 1 teaspoon cumin powder
- ½ teaspoon cinnamon powder
- ½ teaspoon guajillo chili powder Avocado, cilantro & jalapeno, all chopped

DIRECTIONS:

1. Season the chicken with salt & pepper & put the chicken in a pan with coconut oil & brown the pieces of chicken.
2. Transfer the chicken to a cooking pan. Sauté the onion & garlic in the pan & then move it to the cooking pan. Put in the chili peppers, tomatoes, almond butter, dark chocolate, salt & spices to the cooking pan.
3. Cook for 4-6 hrs on low until the chicken is tender.
4. Top with cilantro, avocado & jalapeno.

8. Raspberry Sorbet

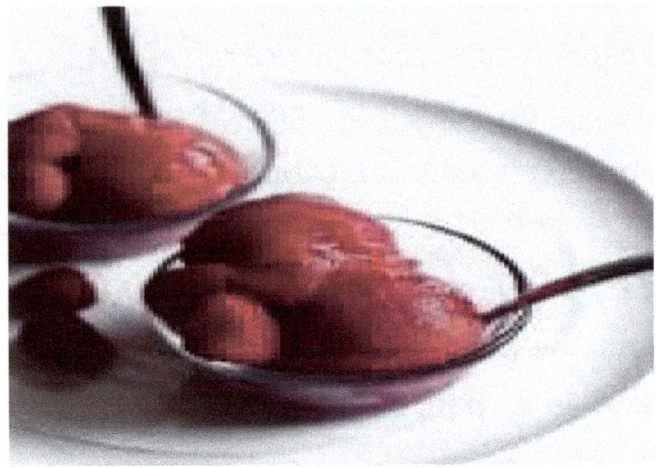

Prep Time: 20 Mins | Cooking Time: 40 Mins | Serve: 3

INGREDIENTS:

- 1 cup water
- 1 teaspoon low-or no-sugar-needed fruit pectin
  ⅛ teaspoon salt
- 1¼ pounds (4 cups) fresh or frozen raspberries
- ½ cup (3½ ounces) plus 2 tablespoons sugar
- ¼ cup light
- Corn syrup

DIRECTIONS:

1. Heat water, pectin, and salt in a medium saucepan over medium-high heat, occasionally stirring, until pectin has fully dissolved, about 5 minutes.
2. Remove saucepan from heat and let the mixture cool slightly for about 10 minutes.
3. Process raspberries, sugar, corn syrup, and cooled water mixture in blender or food processor until smooth, about 30 seconds.
4. Strain mixture through a fine-mesh strainer, pressing on solids to extract as much liquid as possible. Transfer 1 cup mixture to small bowl and place remaining mixture in a large bowl.
5. Cover both bowls with plastic wrap. Place a large bowl in the refrigerator and a small bowl in the freezer and chill for at least 4 hours or up to 24 hours. (Small bowl of the base will freeze solid.)
3. Remove mixtures from refrigerator and freezer.
6. Scrape frozen base from the small bowl into a large bowl of the base. Stir occasionally until the frozen base has fully dissolved.

7. Transfer mixture to ice cream machine and churn until mixture has the consistency of thick milkshake and color lightens, 15 to 25 minutes.
8. Transfer sorbet to an airtight container, pressing firmly to remove any air pockets, and freeze until firm, at least 2 hours or up to 5 days. Let sorbet sit at room temperature for 5 minutes before serving.

9. Mexican Coffee

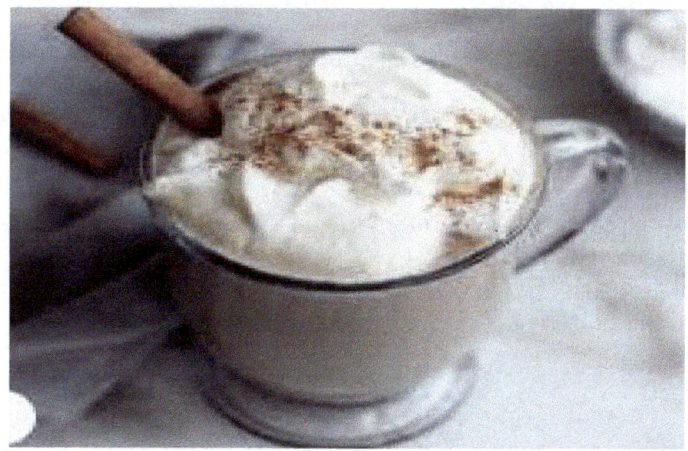

Prep Time: 20 Mins | Cooking Time: 10 Mins | Serve: 3

INGREDIENTS:

- 6 ounces (170 ml) brewed coffee
- 2 to 3 tbsps. (28 to 45 ml) heavy cream
- 2 teaspoons Splenda
- 2 drops blackstrap molasses*
- Tiny pinch ground cinnamon
- Tiny pinch ground cloves

DIRECTIONS:

1. It helps to keep your blackstrap in a squeeze bottle. I buy my blackstrap in bulk from my health food store & keep it in one of those "honey bears."
2. Pour the coffee & stir in the cream, Splenda, & molasses. Sprinkle the spices over the top & serve.

10. Café coffee

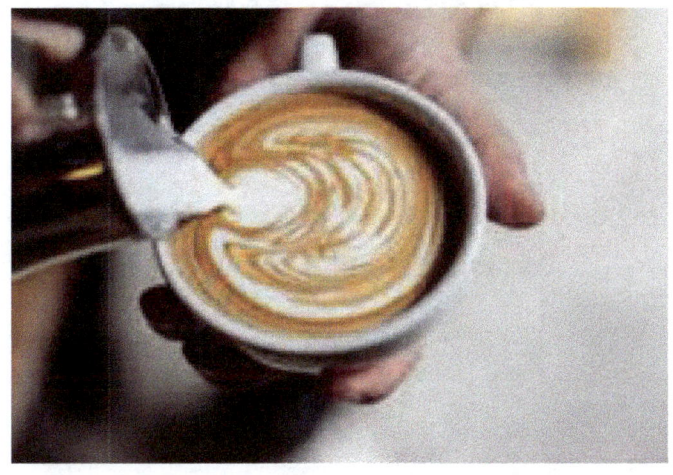

Prep Time: 20 Mins | Cooking Time: 10 Mins | Serve: 3

INGREDIENTS:

- 6 ounces (170 ml) brewed coffee
- 2 tbsps. (30 g) sugar-free chocolate coffee flavoring syrup 2 tbsps. (28 ml) heavy cream
- Tiny pinch ground cinnamon

DIRECTIONS:

1. Pour the coffee, stir in the chocolate syrup & heavy cream, dust the cinnamon over the top, & serve.

11. Chocolate Orange Coffee with cake

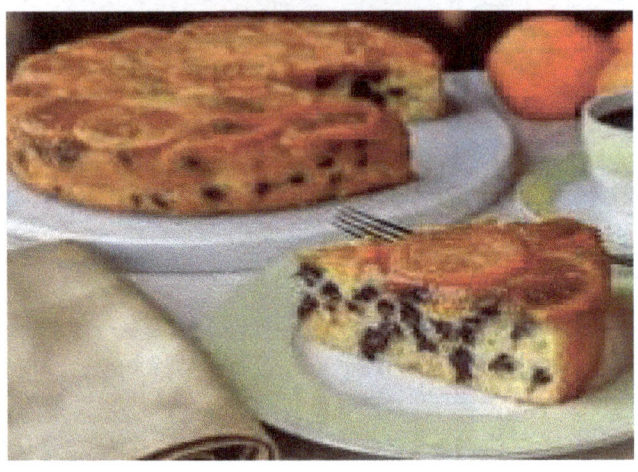

Prep Time: 20 Mins | Cooking Time: 10 Mins | Serve: 3

INGREDIENTS:

- 6 ounces (170 ml) brewed coffee
- 1 tbsp. (15 g) sugar-free chocolate coffee flavoring syrup
- 1 or 2 drops orange extract

DIRECTIONS:

1. Pour the coffee & stir in the syrup & the extract. That's all!

12. Keto Turkey Stir Fry

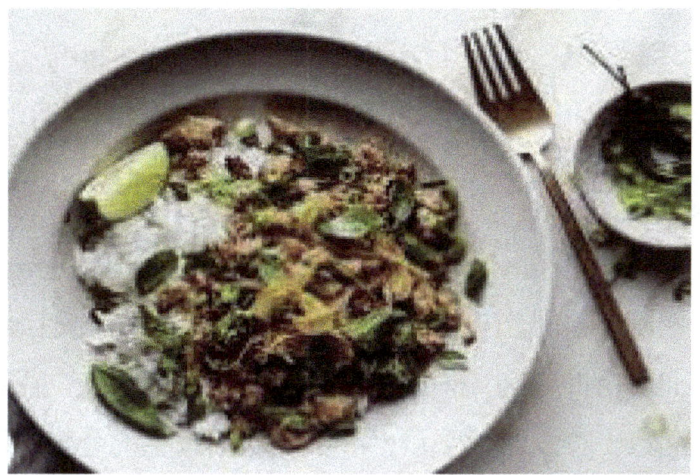

Prep Time: 20 Mins | Cooking Time: 40 Mins | Serve: 4

INGREDIENTS:

- 1 ½ pound (680 grams) boneless turkey tenderloin, sliced very thinly 3 to 4 tbsps. (45 to 60 ml) olive oil
- 1 medium onion, sliced
- 1 medium green pepper, cut into strips
- ¼ cup (60 ml) dry white wine
- ¼ cup (60 ml) lemon juice
- 1 can (2.25 ounces, or 70 grams) sliced ripe olives, drained
- 2 Tsps. minced garlic or 4 cloves garlic, crushed
- 1 Tsp. dried oregano

- 2 Tsps. chicken bouillon concentrate guar or xanthan
- 4 tbsps. (16 grams) fresh chopped parsley

DIRECTIONS:

1. In a large pan or wok, start stir-frying the turkey in olive oil on high heat. When it's about half-done (half the pink is gone), put in the onion & pepper. Continue stir-frying until all the pink is gone from the turkey.
2. put in the wine, lemon juice, olives, garlic, oregano, & bouillon & let the whole thing cook, stirring now & then, for another 3 to 4 mins or until the veggies are tender-crisp.
3. Thicken the pan juices slightly with the guar or xanthan. Turn off the burner, stir in the parsley, & serve.

13. Chicken Asparagus Stir-Fry

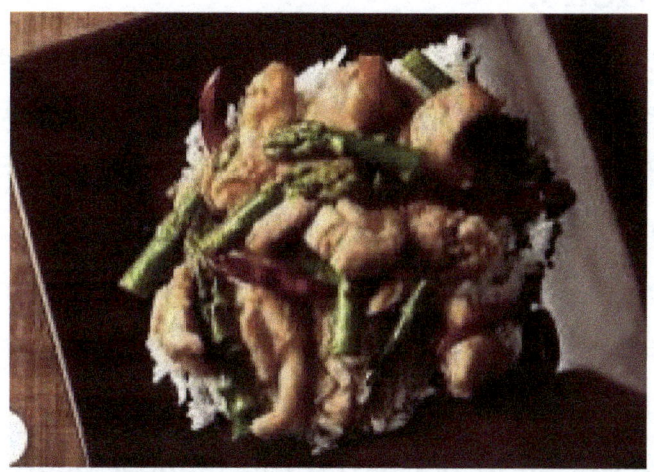

Prep Time: 20 Mins | Cooking Time: 40 Mins | Serve: 3

INGREDIENTS:

- 1 pound (455 grams) asparagus
- 1 medium onion
- 8 ounces (225 grams) canned sliced water chestnuts, drained
- ¼ cup (60 ml) dry sherry
- ¼ cup (60 ml) soy sauce
- 1 Tsp. minced garlic, crushed
- 1 ½ pound (680 grams) boneless, skinless chicken breast, sliced into thin strips
- ¼ cup (60 ml) oil

- Guar or xanthan

DIRECTIONS:

1. Snap the ends off the asparagus where they break naturally & slice diagonally into ½-inch (1.3 cm) lengths. Slice the onion into thin half-rounds.
2. Open the water chestnuts & drain them. Mix together the sherry, soy sauce, & garlic & have it sitting by the stove.
3. Heat the oil in a wok on the highest heat. put in the chicken & stir-fry for 2 to 3 mins or until about half the pink is gone. put in the asparagus & onion & continue stir-frying until the chicken is cooked through.
4. put in the water chestnuts & the sherry batter, stir to combine, & let the whole thing simmer for another 2 to 4 mins or until the asparagus is bright green & tender-crisp.
5. Thicken the juices just a little with the guar or xanthan & serve.

14. Sea Bass with Tapenade Cream Sauce

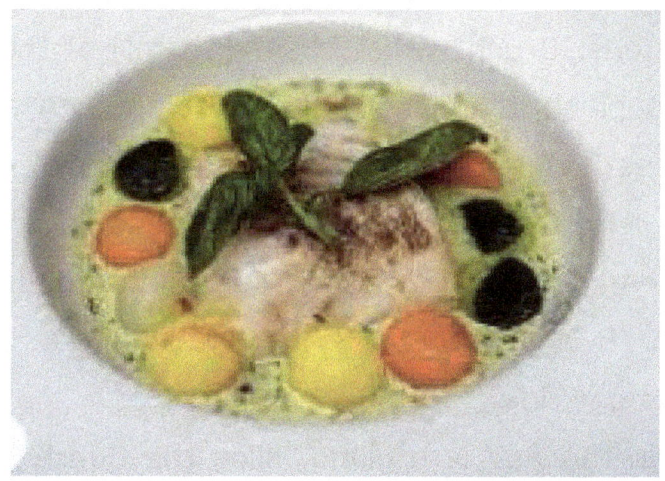

Prep Time: 20 Mins | Cooking Time: 40 Mins | Serve: 3

INGREDIENTS:

- 12 ounces (340 grams) sea bass fillet
- 3 tbsps. (45 ml) olive oil
- ¼ medium onion
- ½ Tsp. minced garlic or 1 clove garlic, crushed
- 2 tbsps. (16 grams) tapenade
- 1 tbsp. (15 ml) balsamic vinegar
- 1 Tsp. lemon juice
- 3 tbsps. (45 ml) heavy cream
- Salt & pepper

DIRECTIONS:

1. If the bass is in one piece, cut it into two equal portions. Brush with 1 tbsp. (15 ml) of the olive oil & place it under a broiler set on High, 3 or 4 inches (7.5 to 10 cm) from the heat.
2. The length of time the fish will need to broil will depend on its thickness. I use fillets about 1 ½-inch (3.8 cm) thick, & they take about 5 to 6 mins per side.
3. While the fish is broiling, slice the quarter-onion in half lengthwise & then slice as thinly as possible. Place the remaining olive oil in a medium-size pan over medium heat & put in the onion & garlic.
4. Sauté together for 3 to 4 mins. put in the tapenade, stir in, & sauté for a few more mins. (Remember that somewhere in here, you'll need to turn the fish!) Now, stir the vinegar & lemon juice into the batter in your pan & let it cook down for 1 to 2 mins.
5. Stir in the cream & let the whole thing cook down for another min.

6. When the fish is ready, transfer it on two serving plates. Salt & pepper the sauce to taste, spoon over the fish, & then serve.

15. Keto Chinese Breakfast Chaffle

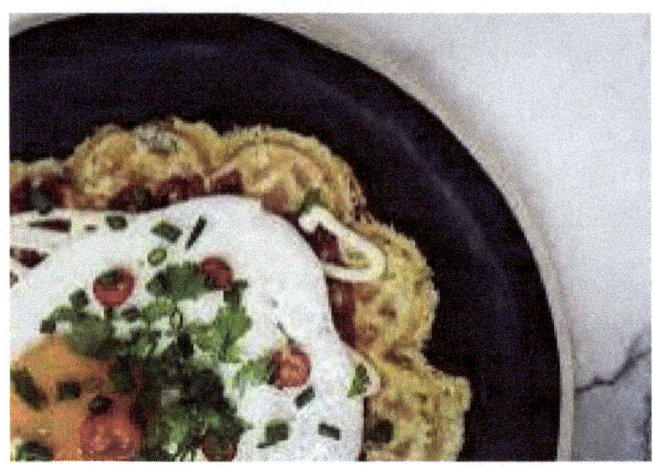

Prep Time: 25Mins | Cooking Time: 35 Mins | Serve: 3

INGREDIENTS:
- Savoury Pancake
- 1 extra-large egg
- 2 cups of grated/grated tasty cheese
- 2 tablespoons spring onions /
- 1.5 teaspoons of coconut flour or 2 tablespoons of almond flour
- Salt and pepper to taste
- 1 fried egg
- mayonnaise
- Sugar-free BBQ sauce

- Fresh cilantro

DIRECTIONS:
1. First, preheat your waffle iron and mix all the ingredients for the chaffle in a small bowl.
2. Then, pour the ingredients from the chaffle into the wafer pan and spread them carefully over the bottom.
3. Now cook until the chaffle is cooked and brown.
4. And carefully remove on a serving plate.
5. To present
6. Serve hot topped with a fried egg.

16. Chicken Bites With Chaffles

Prep Time: 10 Mins | Cooking Time: 25 Mins | Serve: 3

INGREDIENTS:
- 1 chicken fillet cut into 2 x 5 cm pieces
- 1 egg, beaten
- 1/4 cup of almond flour
- 2 tablespoons. onion powder
- 2 tablespoons. garlic powder
- 1 tablespoon. dried oregano
- 1 tablespoon. paprika powder
- 1 tablespoon. salt
- 1/2 tablespoon. black pepper
- 2 tablespoons. avocado oil

DIRECTIONS:
1. Mix all dry components in a large bowl and mix well.
2. put the eggs in a separate bowl.
3. Dip piece of chicken in the egg and then in the dry ingredients.

4. Heat oil in 10-inch skillet, add oil.
5. Once the avocado oil is hot, put the coated chicken nuggets in a skillet and fry for 6-8 mins until tender and golden brown.
6. Serve with chaffles and raspberries.
7. To enjoy!

17. Fish With Chaffle Bites

Prep Time: 20 Mins | Cooking Time: 45 Mins | Serve: 5

INGREDIENTS:

- 1 pound cod fillets, cut into 4 slices
- 1 tablespoon. sea salt
- 1 tablespoon. garlic powder
- 1 egg, beaten
- 1 cup of almond flour
- 2 tablespoons. avocado oil

Chaffle Ingredients:

- 2 eggs
- 1/2 cup of cheddar cheese
- 2 tablespoons. almond flour
- ½ tablespoon. Italian spices

DIRECTIONS:

1. mix the ingredients of the chaffle in a bowl and make 4 squares
2. put the chaffles in a preheated chaffle maker.

3. Mix the salt, pepper, and garlic powder in a mixing bowl.
4. Toss the cod cubes through this batter and let stand for 10 mins.
5. Then dip each slice of cod in the egg batter and then in the almond flour.
6. Heat oil in a skillet and fish cubes for about 2-3 mins, until cooked and brown
7. Present on chaffles and enjoy!

18. Cheddar & Herb Chaffle (Keto Low Carb)

Prep Time: 30 Mins | Cooking Time: 40 Mins | Serve: 5

INGREDIENTS:

- 2 eggs
- 113 g grated aged cheddar cheese
- 2 teaspoon almond flour
- 1 teaspoon of Italian herbal seasoning
- 1/4 teaspoon baking powder
- 1/4 teaspoon of salt

DIRECTIONS:

1. Firstly, preheat a waffle iron and spray it lightly with cooking spray.
2. Beat the eggs, cheese, Italian herbs, baking powder and salt well together.
3. Then pour half of the batter into the waffle iron and cook for 3-4 mins, until lightly browned and cooked through.
4. Carefully remove the wafer and repeat with the remaining batter.

5. Let them cool for 2 mins (to get crisper).
6. Present and appreciate!

19. Chaffles With Keto Ice Cream

Prep Time: 35 Mins | Cooking Time: 45 Mins | Serve: 5

INGREDIENTS:

- 2 eggs
- 113 g grated aged cheddar cheese
- 2 teaspoon almond flour
- 1 teaspoon of Italian herbal seasoning
- 1/4 teaspoon baking powder
- 1/4 teaspoon of salt

DIRECTIONS:

1. Firstly preheat the waffle iron.
2. Mix all ingredients except for the ice cream in a bowl.
3. Open the iron and add half of the batter. Close and cook until crispy, 7 mins.
4. Put the chaffle on a plate and make a second with the remaining batter.
5. Add a measure of low-carb ice cream to each chaffle, fold in crescents and enjoy.

20. Vanilla Mozzarella Chaffles

Prep Time: 15 Mins | Cooking Time: 40 Mins | Serve: 6

INGREDIENTS:
- 1 organic egg, beaten
- 1 teaspoon of organic vanilla extract
- 1 tablespoon of almond flour
- 1 teaspoon of organic baking powder
- Pinch of ground cinnamon
- 1 cup mozzarella cheese, shredded

DIRECTIONS:

1. Firstly, preheat a mini waffle iron and then grease it.
2. Put the egg and vanilla extract in a bowl and beat until well blended.
3. Add the flour, baking powder, and cinnamon and mix well.
4. Add the mozzarella cheese and stir to mix.
5. Put the egg and mozzarella cheese in a small bowl and stir to mix.

6. Put half of the batter in the preheated waffle iron and bake for about 5 mins or until golden brown.
7. Repeat food with the remaining batter.
8. Present warm.

21. Chili's Molten Lava Cake

Prep Time: 20 Mins | Cooking Time: 40 Mins | Serve: 6

INGREDIENTS:
- 5 Tbsps. butter
- 3.5 ounces dark chocolate
- 2 extra-large eggs
- 1 extra-large egg yolk
- 3 Tsps. sugar
- 1 Tsp. vanilla extract
- 3 Tbsps. flour
- 2 Tsps. cocoa powder
- 1 Tsp. salt

DIRECTIONS:
1. Preheat the oven to 425°F.
2. Melt the butter & chocolate together in the microwave for 2-3 mins on medium heat. Stir to combine.

3. In a large mixing bowl, whisk together the eggs, sugar & vanilla until the mixture is light yellow in color & the sugar is dissolved.
4. Stir the warm chocolate mixture into the egg mixture & whisk until combined. Sift in the flour, cocoa, & salt. Fold in with a spatula until combined.
5. Spoon into 4 buttered 5-ounce ramekins, & tap on the table to settle any air bubbles. Refrigerate for 30 mins.
6. Place the ramekins in a baking dish & add water to the dish until it is halfway up the sides—Bake for 10 Mins.

22. Cracker Barrel Banana Pudding

Prep Time: 15 Mins | Cooking Time: 40 Mins | Serve: 8

INGREDIENTS:

- 1½ quarts milk
- 1¼ cups liquid egg substitute
- 11/8 cups flour
- 1 cup vanilla extract
- 1¼ cups sugar
- 12 ounces vanilla wafers
- 1¾ peeled bananas
- 1 (8-ounce) container Cool Whip

DIRECTIONS:

1. Heat the milk in a saucepan to 170°F.
2. In a bowl, mix the eggs, flour, vanilla, & sugar.
3. Add the sugar mixture to the milk in the pan.
4. Cook for 10–12 mins until it becomes custard-like, stirring constantly.
5. Spread the wafers on the bottom of the baking pan.

6. Slice the bananas & place them over the wafers.
7. Pour the custard over the wafers & bananas.
8. Let cool & add Cool Whip to the top.

23. Cracker Barrel Carrot Cake

Prep Time: 15 Mins | Cooking Time: 40 Mins | Serve: 6

INGREDIENTS:
- 3 cups flour
- 2 Tsps. baking powder
- 2 Tsps. baking soda
- ½ Tsp. salt
- 2 Tsps. ground cinnamon
- 1 Tsp. ground nutmeg
- 1 Tsp. ground cloves
- 1¼ cups vegetable oil
- 1½ cups sugar
- 1 cup brown sugar
- 2 Tsps. vanilla
- 3 eggs
- 1 cup crushed pineapple
- 1 cup finely chopped walnuts
- ½ cup shredded coconut
- 2 cups shredded carrots
- ½ cup raisins

- Cream Cheese Frosting
- 8 ounces cream cheese
- 1 cup room-temperature butter
- 1 Tsp. vanilla
- 2 cups powdered sugar
- 1 cup chopped pecans for garnish

DIRECTIONS:

1. Preheat the oven to 350°F.
2. Mix together flour, baking powder, baking soda, salt, cinnamon, nutmeg, & cloves. Set aside.
3. In a large bowl, using a beater, mix the oil, sugars, vanilla, & eggs until smooth & fluffy. Add the pineapple, walnuts, coconut, carrots, & raisins & blend well. Gradually add the flour mixture half at a time until blended through.
4. Pour the batter into a greased & floured 9" × 13" pan & bake for about 40–50 mins. Test with toothpick for doneness.
5. To make the frosting, blend the cream cheese & butter until it is light & fluffy. Add the vanilla & a little powdered sugar at a time until all has been well blended. Turn the mixer on high & beat until frosting is light & fluffy.

6. Spread the frosting over the cooled cake & sprinkle with pecans

24. Cracker Barrel Cherry Chocolate Cobbler

Prep Time: 15 Mins | Cooking Time: 20 Mins | Serve: 8

INGREDIENTS:
- 1½ cups flour
- ½ cup sugar
- 2 Tsps. baking powder
- ½ Tsp. salt
- ¼ cup butter
- 6 ounces semisweet chocolate morsels
- 1 cup milk
- 1 egg
- 1 (21-ounce) can cherry pie filling
- ½ cup finely chopped peanuts

DIRECTIONS:
1. Preheat the oven to 350°F.
2. In a large bowl, combine flour, sugar, baking powder, salt, & butter. Cut with a pastry blender until the crumbs are the size of large peas.

3. Melt the chocolate morsels in the microwave for 2-3 mins on medium. Add the milk & egg & mix well.
4. Blend the chocolate into the flour mixture.
5. Spread the cherry pie filling in the bottom of a 2-quart casserole.
6. Drop the chocolate batter randomly over the cherries & sprinkle the top with chopped nuts.
7. Bake in the oven for 40-45 mins.

25. Golden Corral Bread Pudding

Prep Time: 10 Mins | Cooking Time: 40 Mins | Serve: 4

INGREDIENTS:
- Bread Pudding
- 2 cups milk
- 1 cup butter
- 2 eggs
- 1/3 cup brown sugar
- ¼ Tsp. salt
- 1 Tsp. cinnamon
- 3 cups cubed French bread
- White Sauce
- 1 cup milk
- 2 Tbsps. butter
- ½ cup sugar
- 1 Tsp. vanilla
- 1 Tbsp. flour
- Dash of salt

DIRECTIONS:
1. Preheat the oven to 350°F.
2. In a saucepan over medium, heat the milk & butter together. Remove & set aside.
3. In a large mixing bowl, beat the eggs & add the brown sugar, salt & cinnamon. Let the milk cool for 30 mins then add it to the egg mixture, making sure that the egg mixture does not curdle.
4. Add the bread cubes & stir carefully; do not beat.
5. Place the mixture in an 8" × 11" well-oiled pan & bake for about 40 mins, until a toothpick inserted into the middle comes out clean. Set aside.
6. Mix all the sauce ingredients together & bring to a boil in a pan for 3–4 mins, stirring constantly. Pour about ½ the mixture on the warm bread pudding & place the remainder of the sauce in a serving bowl for those who desire a little extra.

26. Olive Garden Apple Carmelina

Prep Time: 20 Mins | Cooking Time: 40 Mins | Serve: 6

INGREDIENTS:

Filling

- 2 (20-ounce) cans drained sliced apples
- 1 cup sugar
- 1 Tsp. apple pie spice
- ¼ cup brown sugar
- ¼ cup flour
- ¼ Tsp. salt

Topping

- ¾ cup flour
- ¼ Tsp. salt
- 1 cup light brown sugar
- ¼ cup sugar
- 5 Tbsps. softened butter

DIRECTIONS:

1. Preheat the oven to 350°F.
2. Mix all the ingredients for the filling together in a bowl & stir well.
3. Pour the mixture into a lightly buttered 8" × 8" baking dish.
4. Create the topping in a separate bowl by adding the flour, salt, & sugars & blending well. Work in the butter. The mixture should look like a coarse meal.
5. Sprinkle over the apples & bake for 30–35 mins.

27. Starbucks Tarragon Chicken Salad

Prep Time: 15 Mins | Cooking Time: 20 Mins | Serve: 6

INGREDIENTS:

- ¼ cup mayonnaise
- 1 Tbsp. fresh chopped tarragon
- 1 Tsp. lemon juice
- 2 cups ½" cubed cooked chicken
- 1 cup finely chopped dried cranberries
- 1 stalk finely chopped celery
- 1 Tbsp. finely chopped red onion

DIRECTIONS:

1. In a small bowl, create the dressing by combining the mayonnaise, tarragon, & lemon juice.
2. Mix well.
3. In a medium bowl, add the chicken, cranberries, celery, & onion & lightly toss to mix.
4. Add the dressing & mix well.

28. Steak'n Shake Frisco Melt

Prep Time: 15 Mins | Cooking Time: 40 Mins | Serve: 8

INGREDIENTS:
- 3 racks pork baby back ribs
- 1 cup ketchup
- ¼ cup apple cider vinegar
- 3 Tbsps. dark brown sugar
- 3 Tbsps. Worcestershire sauce
- 1 Tsp. liquid smoke
- 1 Tsp. salt

DIRECTIONS:
1. Put the ribs in a large pot with enough water to cover them. Bring the water to a boil, reduce heat, & cover. Simmer for 1 hour, or until ribs are fork-tender.
2. Mix all the remaining ingredients together in a medium pan. Bring to a boil, reduce heat, & simmer uncovered. Cook for 30 mins, stirring often, or until the sauce is slightly thickened.

3. Heat the broiler. Place the ribs meat-side down on the broiler pan; brush the ribs with half the sauce.
4. Broil 4"–5" from heat source for 6–7 mins. Turn the ribs over & brush with the remaining sauce.
5. Broil 6–7 mins longer, or until the edges are slightly charred.

29. Applebee's Garlic & Peppercorn Fried Shrimp

Prep Time: 10 Mins | Cooking Time: 40 Mins | Serve: 8

INGREDIENTS:

- 1 pound (61–90) thawed shrimp
- Vegetable oil, as needed
- ½ cup flour
- ¼ Tsp. salt
- 2 Tsps. divided fresh cracked black pepper
- 1 Tsp. garlic powder
- Tsp. paprika 1 Tsp. sugar
- 2 eggs
- 1 cup bread crumbs

DIRECTIONS:

1. Clean & peel the shrimp. Leave the tails on.
2. Fill a fryer 2"–3" deep with oil & heat to 350°F.
3. In a bowl, combine the flour, salt, 1 Tsp. pepper, garlic powder, paprika, & sugar.
4. In another bowl, beat eggs slightly.

5. In a third bowl, mix the bread crumbs & 1 Tsp. pepper.
6. Coat the shrimp with flour mixture, then eggs, then bread crumb mixture, being careful to shake off the excess between steps & not overcoat.
7. Fry for 2-3 mins, or until golden brown.

30. Applebee's Garlic Mashed Potatoes

Prep Time: 20 Mins | Cooking Time: 40 Mins | Serve: 6

INGREDIENTS:
- 4 whole cloves of garlic
- 2 pounds red potatoes
- ½ cup milk
- 1 cup heavy cream
- 3 Tbsps. butter
- Salt & black pepper, to taste

DIRECTIONS:
1. Preheat the oven to 400°F.
2. Place garlic cloves on a sheet of heavy-duty aluminum foil. Wrap the garlic tightly & roast for approximately 45 mins, or until soft. Unwrap the garlic & let it cool until touchable.
3. Wash & rinse the potatoes. It is not necessary to peel the potatoes unless you desire.

4. Place the potatoes in a large pot & boil for 20 mins. Remove them from the heat & drain them in a colander.
5. Peel the garlic cloves. Combine them with the potatoes & all other ingredients & mash with a potato masher.

31. Applebee's Tequila Lime Chicken

Prep Time: 15 Mins | Cooking Time: 20 Mins | Serve: 8

INGREDIENTS:

- 1 cup lime juice
- ¼ cup tequila
- 1 boneless skinless chicken breast
- 1 Tbsp. salsa
- 3 Tbsps. ranch dressing
- 1 cup tortilla chips
- 1 cup shredded Cheddar jack cheese

DIRECTIONS:

1. Pour the lime juice & tequila into a sealable plastic bag. Add the chicken & allow it to marinate for 2–3 hours.
2. Preheat the grill to medium-high heat & also preheat the broiler.
3. Remove the chicken from the marinade. Grill it for 10 mins, or until thoroughly cooked.
4. Combine salsa & ranch dressing in a small bowl.

5. Scatter the tortilla chips on an oven-safe plate.
6. Place the chicken on top of the tortilla chips.
7. Pour the dressing mixture over the chicken.
8. Cover the chicken with the cheese.
9. Place the chicken under the broiler until cheese is melted.

32. Buca di Beppo Chicken Marsala

Prep Time: 15 Mins | Cooking Time: 40 Mins | Serve: 6

INGREDIENTS:

- 4 boneless skinless chicken breasts
- 1 cup flour
- Salt & pepper, to taste
- 1 Tbsp. oregano
- 2 Tbsps. olive oil
- 1 Tbsp. butter
- 2 cups Marsala wine
- 3 cups chicken stock
- 1¼ cups sliced fresh mushrooms
- 4 minced garlic cloves
- 1 (16-ounce) package cooked linguini or spaghetti

DIRECTIONS:

1. Place chicken breasts one at a time between 2 sheets of waxed paper. Pound until they are about ¼ " thick.

2. In a small bowl, combine flour, salt, pepper, & oregano.
3. Dredge chicken in flour until coated thoroughly.
4. Heat the olive oil & butter in a large skillet.
5. Fry chicken breasts until they are almost fully cooked, about 3 mins on each side. Remove from pan.
6. Deglaze the pan with the wine. Make sure to scrape all the brown bits on the bottom of the pan & mix with the wine.
7. Add chicken stock, mushrooms, & garlic. Cook the broth on medium-high for 10 mins, or until the sauce has been reduced by half.
8. Add chicken breasts back into the pan & cook for another 10 mins. The sauce should become thick.
9. Serve over pasta.

33. Buca di Beppo Penne Cardinale

Prep Time: 10 Mins | Cooking Time: 40 Mins | Serve: 6

INGREDIENTS:
- 1 pound chicken tenders
- ¾ cup olive oil
- cup green onions ¼ cup chopped garlic 1 Tsp. salt
- 2 Tsp. crushed red pepper flakes
- 1 cup white wine
- 1¼ cups quartered artichokes
- 1½ cups cream
- 2 pats butter
- 1¾ pounds cooked penne pasta
- 1 cup grated Romano cheese

DIRECTIONS:
1. Cut the chicken in half lengthwise.
2. In a large sauté pan, heat olive oil & sauté onions & garlic for 3-4 mins, until slightly browned.

3. Add the chicken, salt, & red pepper. Cook for an additional 3–4 mins until the chicken is done.
4. Deglaze the pan with white wine. Add artichokes & cream. Reduce the sauce until it starts to thicken. Cook for 4–5 mins.
5. Remove the pan from the heat & incorporate the butter. Toss with the cooked penne & then the Romano cheese.

34. Buca di Beppo Chicken Saltimbocca

Prep Time: 15 Mins | Cooking Time: 40 Mins | Serve: 4

INGREDIENTS:
- 1 Tbsp. salt
- 4 (5-ounce) chicken breasts
- 1 Tbsp. chopped fresh sage
- 4 thin slices of prosciutto ham
- 3 ounces olive oil
- 1 ounce all-purpose flour
- 4 ounces white wine
- 5 ounces artichoke hearts, quartered
- 2 ounces fresh lemon juice
- 2 ounces heavy cream
- 1 Tbsp. butter
- 1 ounce capers

DIRECTIONS:
1. Lightly salt the chicken breasts & sprinkle evenly with sage.

2. Place the prosciutto on top of the chicken & pound it into the breast until the thickness of the chicken measures 3/8".
3. In a sauté pan, heat the olive oil over medium heat.
4. Lightly flour the flattened chicken.
5. Place chicken into the pan, Prosciutto side down. Brown one side, turn & brown the other side.
6. Drain off excess oil, & deglaze with white wine. Add the artichokes, lemon juice, cream, & butter & cook until sauce is thickened.
7. On a large platter, place the chicken breasts topped with reduced sauce & garnish with capers.

35. Carino's Angel Hair with Artichokes

Prep Time: 20 Mins | Cooking Time: 20 Mins | Serve: 8

INGREDIENTS:

- 1 Tbsps. extra-virgin olive oil
- 1 Tsp. fresh chopped garlic
- 14 large shrimp
- 1 cup quartered artichoke hearts
- 1 cup diced Roma tomatoes
- 1 cup chopped black olives
- 4 Tbsps. capers Salt & pepper, to taste
- ¼ cup chopped fresh basil
- 1 pound angel hair pasta, cooked
- 2 Tbsps. shredded Parmesan
- Fresh chopped parsley, for garnish

DIRECTIONS:

1. In a sauté pan on medium, add olive oil, garlic, shrimp, & artichokes. Let shrimp cook & let the garlic turn a golden color to develop flavor (about 3–4 mins).

2. Add tomatoes, black olives, capers, salt, & pepper. Let ingredients thoroughly heat while mixing. Cook 5–6 mins.
3. Remove from the heat & toss in fresh basil.
4. Place cooked pasta in a mound on a service plate & top with ingredients from a sauté pan, then garnish with Parmesan & parsley.

36. Carino's Five Meat Tuscan Pasta

Prep Time: 15 Mins | Cooking Time: 40 Mins | Serve: 8

INGREDIENTS:
- 2 Tbsps. olive oil
- 2 Tsps. chopped garlic
- 1 cup sliced cooked Italian sausage
- 1 cup diced ham
- 1 cup chopped bacon
- ¼ cup chopped pepperoni
- 1 cup diced green bell peppers
- 1 cup diced yellow onions
- Salt & pepper, to taste
- 2½ cups meat sauce
- 1 (16-ounce) box cooked bowtie pasta
- 1 cup shredded Asiago cheese
- 1 cup shredded Parmesan cheese

DIRECTIONS:

1. In a large sauté pan over medium heat, add the olive oil, garlic, sausage, ham, bacon, pepperoni, bell peppers, onions, salt, & pepper.
2. Sauté 8–10 mins until the bacon is cooked & peppers & onions are soft.
3. Add meat sauce & pasta & toss together.
4. Place the pasta on a serving plate & garnish with Asiago & Parmesan cheeses.

37. Carino's Grilled Chicken Bowtie Festival

Prep Time: 10 Mins | Cooking Time: 40 Mins | Serve: 6

INGREDIENTS:

- 2 Tbsps. melted butter
- 1/8 cup diced red onion
- 1 Tsp. chopped fresh garlic
- 1 cup diced Roma tomatoes
- 1 cup diced cooked bacon
- 1 cup sliced cooked chicken
- Salt, pepper, & garlic salt, to taste
- 1-ounce heavy cream
- 1/8 cup Asiago cheese
- 1 (16-ounce) jar of Ragu Alfredo sauce
- (16-ounce) box cooked bowtie pasta

DIRECTIONS:

1. In a heated sauté pan, combine butter, onions, garlic, tomatoes, bacon, chicken, salt, pepper, & garlic salt.

2. After 3-4 mins, when the onions turn translucent, add the cream & Asiago.
3. Once the cheese & cream have reduced (about 6-8 mins), add the Alfredo sauce & pasta.
4. Toss & combine well.
5. Allow cooling a few mins for the sauce & cheese to thicken.

38. Cheesecake Factory Jambalaya Pasta

Prep Time: 15 Mins | Cooking Time: 40 Mins | Serve: 4

INGREDIENTS:
- 1 green bell pepper
- 1 red bell pepper
- ½ red onion
- 1 pound boneless, skinless chicken breasts
- 1 stick of butter
- 2 Tsps. Cajun spice mix
- 1 pound linguini pasta
- 1 cup clam juice
- 1 pound peeled fresh medium shrimp
- 1 cup diced tomatoes

DIRECTIONS:
1. Slice the peppers & onions into thin strips & cut the chicken into small pieces.
2. Place the butter in a sauté pan & allow it to melt slightly. Add the spice mix & stir together with the butter.

3. Add the chicken & continue to cook for 4 mins until the chicken is about half done.
4. While the chicken is cooking, cook the pasta until al dente.
5. Pour the clam juice into the pan & add the peppers & onions. Cook for another min, making sure the vegetables are heated through & the chicken is almost done.
6. Add the shrimp & toss the ingredients together. Continue to cook for 3 mins until the shrimp are almost done.
7. Add the tomatoes & continue to cook for 5 more mins until both the shrimp & chicken are thoroughly cooked.
8. Place some pasta into each bowl. Spoon equal portions of the jambalaya mixture over the pasta.

39. Cracker Barrel Baby Carrots

Prep Time: 20 Mins | Cooking Time: 40 Mins | Serve: 8

INGREDIENTS:

- ¼ cup butter
- (1-pound) package washed baby carrots
- 2 Tbsps. water
- 2 Tbsps. brown sugar
- ¼ Tsp. salt

DIRECTIONS:

1. Melt the butter in a saucepan over medium heat.
2. Add the remaining ingredients.
3. Cover & cook on medium-low for 35–20 Mins, stirring twice.

40. Cracker Barrel Corn Bread Dressing

Prep Time: 15 Mins | Cooking Time: 40 Mins | Serve: 8

INGREDIENTS:
- 2/3 cup chopped onion
- 2 cups chopped celery
- 2 cups day-old grated cornbread
- 4 cups day-old grated biscuits
- ¼ cup dried parsley flakes
- 2 Tsps. poultry seasoning
- 2 Tsps. ground sage
- 1 Tsp. coarse-ground pepper
- 1 stick melted butter
- 1 quart plus 1 (14-ounce) can chicken broth

DIRECTIONS:
1. Preheat the oven to 400°F.
2. In a large mixing bowl, mix the onion, celery, cornbread, biscuits, parsley, poultry seasoning, sage, & pepper. Add the butter & blend well.

3. Add chicken broth to dry ingredients & mix well. The dressing should have a wet but not soupy consistency, like a quick-bread batter.
4. Divide the mixture evenly into two 8" pans sprayed with nonstick spray. Bake uncovered for 1 hour, or until lightly brown on the top.

41. Cracker Barrel Country Green Beans

Prep Time: 10 Mins | Cooking Time: 40 Mins | Serve: 6

INGREDIENTS:

- ¼ pound sliced bacon
- (14½-ounce) cans whole green beans
- ½ Tsp. salt
- 1 Tsp. sugar
- ½ Tsp. black pepper
- ¼ diced yellow onion

DIRECTIONS:

1. In a 2-quart saucepan over medium heat, cook the bacon for 10–12 mins until lightly brown but not crisp.
2. When the bacon has browned, add the green beans & liquid from the cans. Add salt, sugar, & pepper & mix well.
3. Place onions on top of the green beans. Cover the saucepan with a lid & bring to a light boil.
4. Turn the heat down to low & simmer for 45 mins.

42. Cracker Barrel Grilled Chicken Tenders

Prep Time: 15 Mins | Cooking Time: 40 Mins | Serve: 4

INGREDIENTS:

- ½ cup Italian dressing
- 1 Tsp. fresh lime juice
- 1½ Tsps. honey
- 1 pound chicken breast tenders

DIRECTIONS:

1. Mix the dressing, lime juice, & honey together.
2. Pour the mixture over the chicken tenders, making sure all the chicken is covered. Marinate for 1 hour in the refrigerator.
3. Grill the chicken to a light golden color, about 2 mins per side.

43. Popeye's Biscuits

Prep Time: 15 Mins | Cooking Time: 40 Mins | Serve: 4

INGREDIENTS:
- 4 cups Bisquick
- 8 ounces sour cream
- 1 cup club soda
- ½ stick butter

DIRECTIONS:
1. Preheat the oven to 400°F.
2. In a large bowl, mix together the Bisquick, sour cream, & club soda. Turn the dough out onto lightly floured wax paper & pat it out flat with your hand. Cut with a biscuit cutter.
3. Place the biscuits in a baking pan.
4. Melt butter in the microwave & pour ½ the butter over the biscuits before you bake them.
5. Bake the biscuits for 15–20 mins.
6. Brush the remainder of the butter over the biscuits as soon as they come out of the oven.

44. Popeye's Cajun Gravy

Prep Time: 20 Mins | Cooking Time: 20 Mins | Serve: 8

INGREDIENTS:
- 1 Tbsp. vegetable oil
- 1 chicken gizzard
- 1 cup ground beef
- 1 cup ground pork
- 2 Tbsps. minced green bell pepper
- 2 cups water
- (14-ounce) can beef broth
- 2 Tbsps. cornstarch
- 1 Tbsp. flour
- 2 Tsps. milk
- 2 Tsps. distilled white vinegar
- 1 Tsp. sugar
- 1 Tsp. salt
- 1 Tsp. coarse-ground black pepper
- ¼ Tsp. cayenne pepper
- 1/8 Tsp. garlic powder
- 1/8 Tsp. onion powder
- Dash dried parsley flakes

DIRECTIONS:
1. Heat the vegetable oil in a large saucepan over medium heat. Sauté the chicken gizzard for 4–5 mins, until cooked. Remove the gizzard from the pan & let cool. Finely mince the gizzard after it has cooled.
2. In a medium bowl, combine the beef & pork. Mix well with your hands.
3. Add the bell pepper to the saucepan & sauté it for 1 min. Add the beef & pork to the pan & cook for 6–8 mins until brown. Mash the meat into tiny pieces as it browns.
4. Add water & beef broth to the saucepan, & immediately whisk in the cornstarch & flour.
5. Add the remaining ingredients & bring to a boil. Reduce the heat & simmer for 30–35 mins, until the gravy is thick.

45. McDonald's Steak, Egg, & Cheese Bagel Sandwich

Prep Time: 15 Mins | Cooking Time: 40 Mins | Serve: 6

INGREDIENTS:
- 1 beef cube steak, cut into 2 pieces
- 2 Tbsps. Worcestershire sauce
- 1½ Tsps. garlic salt
- 1 Tsp. minced onion
- 2 Tbsps. butter
- 2 split bagels
- 2 eggs
- 2 slices American cheese

DIRECTIONS:
1. Place the steaks in a plastic bag with the Worcestershire sauce, garlic salt, & onion.
2. Cook the steak on a George Foreman indoor grill for about 5 mins, or until done. Remove.
3. Butter the insides of the bagel & toast on the grill.

4. Whisk the eggs in a small bowl.
5. Spray a skillet with nonstick spray & cook the eggs.
6. Once the egg has set, fold in half like an omelette & cut into 4 equal pieces.
7. Place the steak on the bottom of a bagel half, add egg & cheese, then top with the other half of the bagel.

46. Starbucks Bran Muffins

Prep Time: 10 Mins | Cooking Time: 40 Mins | Serve: 4

INGREDIENTS:

- 2½ cups flour
- 2 Tsps. baking soda
- 1½ Tsps. salt
- 2 cups crushed bran cereal
- 1 cup chopped dried apple
- 1 cup dried cherries
- 1 cup boiling water
- 1 cup softened unsalted butter
- 1 cup sugar
- 1 cup honey
- 2 large eggs
- 2 cups buttermilk
- 1 cup walnut pieces

DIRECTIONS:

1. Preheat oven to 400°F. Line a muffin tin with baking cups.

2. In a small bowl, stir flour, baking soda, & salt.
3. In another bowl, combine bran cereal & dried fruit with the boiling water.
4. In a large bowl, beat butter until creamy. Gradually beat in sugar, honey, & eggs.
5. Add the buttermilk to the butter mixture & beat in. Then add the flour mixture, then bran mixture, & the walnuts.
6. Divide the batter into the lined muffin tins.
7. Bake muffins for 20 mins.

47. Applebee's Pico de Gallo

Prep Time: 15 Mins | Cooking Time: 40 Mins | Serve: 8

INGREDIENTS:

- 1 cup diced tomatoes
- ½ cup diced red onion
- 1 finely diced jalapeño pepper
- 1/8 cup roughly chopped cilantro leaves
- ½ Tsp. salt
- 1 Tsp. black pepper
- 1 Tsp. garlic powder
- 1 Tsp. salad oil
- 1 Tsp. white vinegar

DIRECTIONS:

1. In a medium bowl, add tomatoes, onion, & jalapeño.
2. Add the cilantro, salt, pepper, garlic powder, oil, & vinegar & mix gently.

3. Store the leftover pico de gallo in the refrigerator for up to 36 hours to add to your favorite dishes & salads.

48. Applebee's Spinach & Artichoke Dip

Prep Time: 15 Mins | Cooking Time: 20 Mins | Serve: 8

INGREDIENTS:

- 1 (14-ounce) can drain & chopped artichoke hearts
- (10-ounce) box frozen chopped spinach
- (10-ounce) jar Alfredo sauce
- 1 cup of shredded Parmesan & Romano cheese blend
- 2 diced Roma tomatoes
- 4 ounces softened cream cheese
- ½ cup shredded mozzarella cheese
- 1 Tsp. fresh minced garlic

DIRECTIONS:

1. Combine all the ingredients in a mixing bowl.
2. Spread the mixture into a small baking dish.
3. Bake in a 350°F oven for 30 mins, or until the cheeses melt.

49. Olive Garden Pasta e Fagioli Soup

Prep Time: 15 Mins | Cooking Time: 40 Mins | Serve: 6

INGREDIENTS:
- 2 pounds ground beef
- 1 chopped onion
- 3 chopped carrots
- 4 stalks chopped celery
- 2 (28-ounce) cans of undrained diced tomatoes
- (16-ounce) can drain red kidney beans
- (16-ounce) can drain white kidney beans
- 3 (10-ounce) cans beef stock
- 3 Tsps. oregano
- 2 Tsps. pepper
- 5 Tsps. parsley
- 1 Tsp. Tabasco sauce (optional)
- (20-ounce) jar spaghetti sauce
- 8 ounces pasta

DIRECTIONS:

1. Brown the beef in a skillet.
2. Drain the fat from beef & add to a slow cooker with everything except the pasta.
3. Cook on low for 7–8 hours or on high for 4–5 hours.
4. During the last 30 mins, add the pasta & cook on high.

50. Olive Garden Pasta Roma Soup

Prep Time: 10 Mins | Cooking Time: 40 Mins | Serve: 4

INGREDIENTS:

- 2 (16-ounce) cans drained garbanzo beans
- 1/3 cup olive oil
- 1 cup julienned carrots
- 1 cup diced onions
- 1 cup diced celery
- ¼ Tsp. minced garlic
- 6 slices cooked bacon
- 1½ cups canned drained, chopped tomatoes
- 1-quart chicken broth
- ½ Tsp. black pepper
- 1/8 Tsp. ground rosemary
- 2 Tbsps. chopped fresh parsley
- 1 cup cooked macaroni

DIRECTIONS:

1. Add the beans to a food processor & pulse on & off until the beans are mashed well.

2. Heat the oil in a large soup pot. Add the carrots, onions, celery, & garlic & sauté for 5 mins on medium heat.
3. Add the remaining ingredients except for pasta to the pot. Bring everything to a boil. Reduce heat to a simmer & cook for 20 mins, stirring occasionally.
4. Add the pasta to the finished soup & serve immediately.

51. Olive Garden Seafood Pasta Chowder

Prep Time: 20 Mins | Cooking Time: 40 Mins | Serve: 4

INGREDIENTS:

- 6 ounces small shells or bowtie pasta
- 3 ounces crab meat
- 6 Tbsps. butter
- ½ pound sliced fresh mushrooms
- (1-ounce) packages Newburg sauce
- 3 cups milk 1½ cups water
- ¼ cup dry white wine
- ¼ cup sliced green onions

DIRECTIONS:

1. Cook the pasta according to the package directions.
2. Sort the crab meat to remove any shell pieces.
3. Melt the butter in a 3-quart saucepan. Add the mushrooms & sauté for 3 mins.
4. Add the Newburg sauce & stir well.

5. Add the milk, water, & wine & stir well until the mixture comes to a boil. Reduce heat & simmer for 5–8 mins, stirring constantly.
6. Add the green onions, pasta, & crab. Stir to combine & heat another 5–10 mins.

52. Olive Garden Zuppa Toscana Soup

Prep Time: 15 Mins | Cooking Time: 20 Mins | Serve: 8

INGREDIENTS:

- 1 pound Italian sausage, crumbled
- 1 pound smoked bacon, chopped
- 1 large chopped onion
- 2 large diced russet baking potatoes
- 2 (14.5-ounce) cans chicken broth
- 1-quart water
- 2 cloves minced garlic Salt & pepper, to taste
- 2 cups chopped kale or Swiss chard
- 1 cup heavy whipping cream

DIRECTIONS:

1. Cook the sausage in a 300°F oven for approximately 30 mins. Drain on paper towels.
2. Brown bacon in a small skillet over medium-high heat. Drain on paper towels.

3. Place the onions, potatoes, broth, water, & garlic in a soup pot. Cook on medium heat for 15 mins or until the potatoes are done.
4. Add the sausage & bacon. Sprinkle in salt & pepper to taste.
5. Simmer for another 10 mins. Turn to low heat.
6. Add the kale & cream. Heat another 5–10 mins.

53. P.F. Chang's Wonton Soup

Prep Time: 10 Mins | Cooking Time: 40 Mins | Serve: 8

INGREDIENTS:

For the Soup

- 4 cups chicken stock
- 2 cubed chicken breast halves without skin
- 1 pound peeled medium shrimp
- 1 cup torn fresh spinach
- 1 cup sliced mushrooms
- 1 (8-ounce) can drained water chestnuts
- 1 Tsp. light brown sugar
- 1 Tbsp. Chinese rice wine or dry sherry
- 2 Tbsps. soy sauce
- 1 Tsp. finely chopped green onion
- 1 Tsp. finely chopped fresh ginger

For the Homemade Wontons

- ½ pound pork, coarsely chopped
- 8 coarsely chopped medium shrimp
- 1 Tsp. light brown sugar
- 1 Tbsp. Chinese rice wine or dry sherry

- Tbsp. soy sauce
- 1 Tsp. finely chopped green onion
- 1 Tsp. finely chopped fresh ginger
- 24 wonton wrappers

DIRECTIONS:

1. Bring the stock to a rolling boil. Add the remaining ingredients. Cook the chicken in the soup for about 10 mins.
2. For the homemade wontons, in a bowl, mix the pork & shrimp with brown sugar, rice wine, soy sauce, green onions, & ginger. Blend well & set aside for 25–30 mins for the flavors to blend.
3. Place 1 Tsp. of the filling in the center of each wonton wrapper. Wet the edges of each wonton with a little water & press them together with your fingers to seal. Fold each wonton over.
4. To cook, add wontons to boiling chicken stock & cook for 4–5 mins. Transfer to individual soup bowls & serve garnished with thinly sliced green onions.

54. Red Lobster Clam Chowder

Prep Time: 15 Mins | Cooking Time: 40 Mins | Serve: 6

INGREDIENTS:

- 2 Tbsps. butter
- 1 Tsp. chopped garlic
- 1 cup diced onions
- ½ cup diced celery
- ½ cup diced leeks
- 2 Tbsps. flour
- 4 cups milk
- 1 cup minced clams with juice
- 1 cup diced potatoes
- 1 Tbsp. salt
- 1 Tsp. thyme
- ½ cup heavy cream

DIRECTIONS:

1. Melt the butter in a soup pot over medium heat. Sauté the garlic, onion, celery, & leeks for 3-4 mins.

2. Remove from the heat, add flour, & mix well.
3. Return to the stove. Add the milk & stir.
4. Drain clams & add the juice to the soup. Bring to a boil, stirring often.
5. Reduce heat to a simmer. Add the potatoes & seasonings. Simmer for 10 mins.
6. Add the clams & simmer for 5–8 mins. Finish by adding the heavy cream.

55. Ruby Tuesday White Chicken Chili

Prep Time: 20 Mins | Cooking Time: 40 Mins | Serve: 8

INGREDIENTS:

- 1 pound great northern beans
- 6 cups chicken stock
- 2 medium chopped onions
- 2 minced garlic cloves
- 6 cups diced cooked chicken
- 1 cup salsa
- 2 seeded & diced jalapeño peppers
- 2 diced chili peppers
- 1½ Tsps. oregano
- 2 Tsps. cumin
- 1 Tsp. cayenne pepper
- 1 Tbsp. vegetable oil Salt, to taste

DIRECTIONS:
1. Soak beans in water overnight.
2. The next day, drain the beans. Add beans, chicken stock, & half the onions & garlic to a large stockpot.
3. Simmer for 2 hours until the beans soften, stirring frequently. Add the chicken & salsa.
4. In a skillet, sauté peppers, spices, & the remaining onions & garlic in oil for 3–4 mins. Add to the chili pot along with salt & pepper.
5. Simmer for 1 more hour.

56. Steak'n Shake Chili

Prep Time: 15 Mins | Cooking Time: 20 Mins | Serve: 4

INGREDIENTS:
- 2 Tbsps. vegetable oil
- 1 small diced onion
- 1½ pounds ground beef
- 1 (10.5-ounce) can Campbell's French onion soup
- Tsp. salt
- 1 Tbsp. chili powder
- 2 Tsps. ground cumin
- 1 Tsp. black pepper
- 2 Tsps. cocoa
- 2 (15-ounce) cans of chili beans
- 1 (6-ounce) can tomato paste
- 1 (8-ounce) can tomato sauce
- 1 cup cola

DIRECTIONS:
1. Place oil, onion, & hamburger in a large stockpot over medium heat.

2. Cook the hamburger for 7-9 mins, until it has browned. Drain the excess oil.
3. Add the onion soup & simmer for a few mins.
4. Add the rest of the ingredients to the pot.
5. Simmer on the stove for 1 hour.

57. T.G.I. Friday's Broccoli Cheese Soup

Prep Time: 10 Mins | Cooking Time: 40 Mins | Serve: 4

INGREDIENTS:
- 4 cups chicken broth
- 1 cup half-and-half
- 1 cup water
- 4 slices American cheese
- 1 cup flour
- 1 Tsp. dried onion flakes
- ¼ Tsp. black pepper
- 4½ cups bite-size broccoli florets

DIRECTIONS:
1. Combine all the ingredients except the broccoli into a large soup pot.
2. Bring to a boil, stirring constantly.
3. Reduce to a simmer.
4. Add the broccoli & simmer for 15 mins, or until the broccoli is tender.
5. Garnish with shredded Cheddar cheese.

58. T.G.I. Friday's French Onion Soup

Prep Time: 15 Mins | Cooking Time: 40 Mins | Serve: 6

INGREDIENTS:

- 2 Tbsps. butter
- 4 medium sliced onions
- 4 cups beef broth
- 1 Tbsp. Worcestershire sauce
- 1 Tsp. black pepper
- Dash of dried thyme
- 1 cup French bread cubes
- ½ cup shredded mozzarella cheese

DIRECTIONS:

1. Melt the butter in a 2-quart saucepan over low heat.
2. Add the onions & cook for 20 mins, stirring occasionally. Add the broth, Worcestershire sauce, pepper, & thyme.
3. Increase the heat to medium-high & bring to a boil.

4. Reduce the heat to low, cover, & simmer for 5 mins.
5. Divide soup into 4 individual serving crocks. Place the bread cubes on top of the soup & then add the cheese.
6. Put the soup bowls under the broiler to melt the cheese until it turns slightly brown.

59. Applebee's Oriental Chicken Salad

Prep Time: 15 Mins | Cooking Time: 40 Mins | Serve: 8

INGREDIENTS:
- 4 frozen breaded chicken tenderloins

Dressing
- 6 Tbsps. honey
- 3 Tbsps. rice wine vinegar
- ½ cup mayonnaise
- 2 Tsps. Dijon mustard
- ¼ Tsp. sesame oil

Salad
- 2 cups chopped green cabbage
- 2 cups chopped red cabbage
- 6 cups chopped romaine lettuce
- 1 shredded carrot
- 2 chopped green onions
- 1 cup toasted sliced almonds
- 2/3 cup chow mein noodles

DIRECTIONS:
1. Preheat the oven & cook chicken tenders according to package directions.
2. Combine all the ingredients for the dressing in a small bowl. Stir well & chill in the refrigerator for 30 mins.
3. Combine all the salad ingredients & toss with the dressing.

Conclusion

This is one of my favorite recipe books! In this, you'll find low-carb swaps and suggestions for replacing your favorite high-carb foods with keto-friendly options like swapping croutons for low-carb cheese crisps. You'll also find ways to do keto on a budget, special occasion keto, dining out meal suggestions, and ways to keep it keto while traveling. I hope you like it!

Lightning Source UK Ltd.
Milton Keynes UK
UKHW020645290621
386332UK00001B/36